When Mom-Mom and Pop-Pop Forget

DEBI MASTRODDI

PAGE PUBLISHING, INC.
Conneaut Lake, PA

First originally published by Page Publishing 2022

ISBN 978-1-6624-6115-6 (pbk)
ISBN 978-1-6624-6116-3 (digital)

Printed in the United States of America

Each day I love to visit you
I sing to you,
"How do you do?"
Then you sing to me,
"I'm doing fine."
And you say to me,
"I have not seen you in some time,"
Even though I know
I was here yesterday
I sing to you,
"How do you do?"
Then you sing to me,
"I'm doing fine."

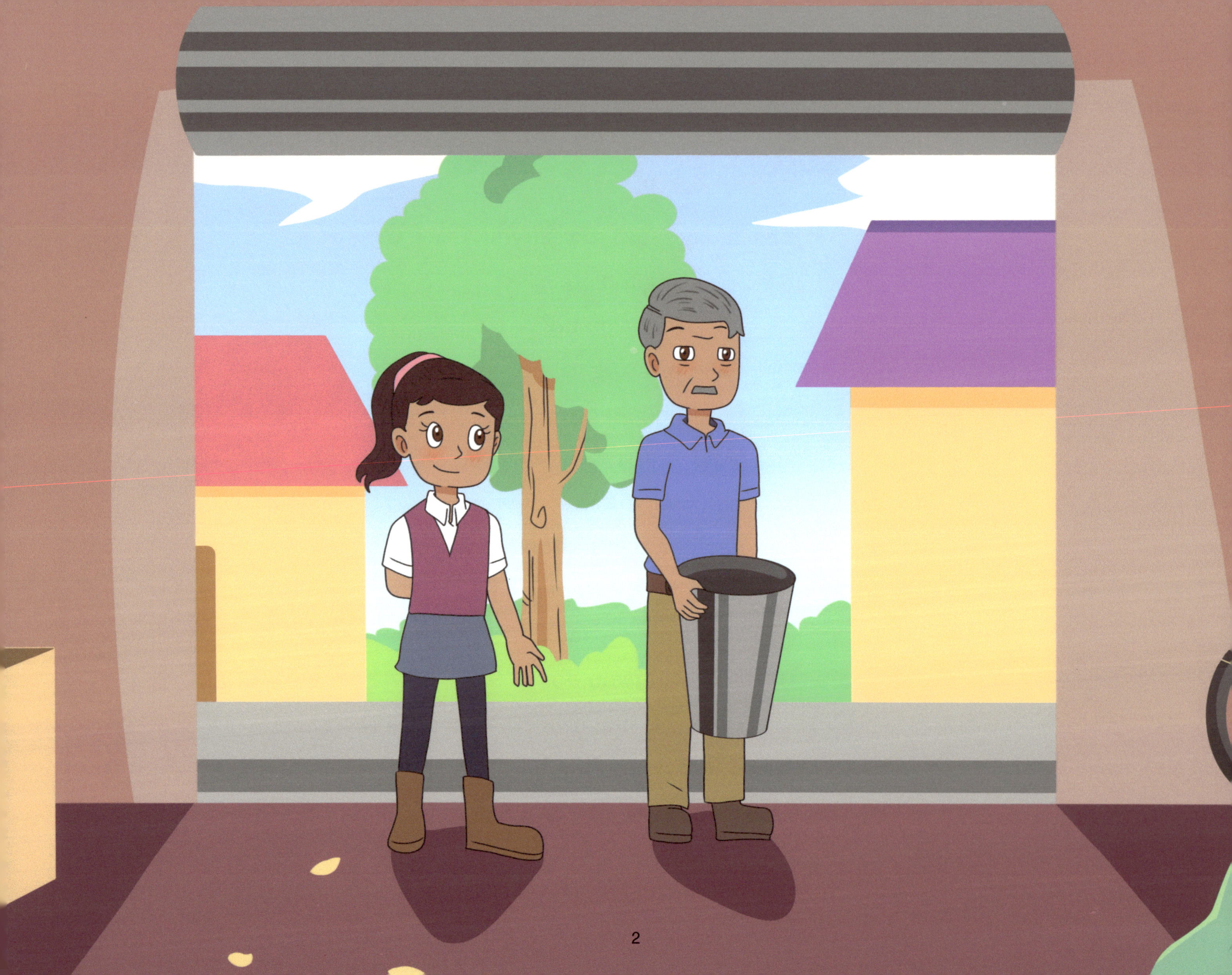

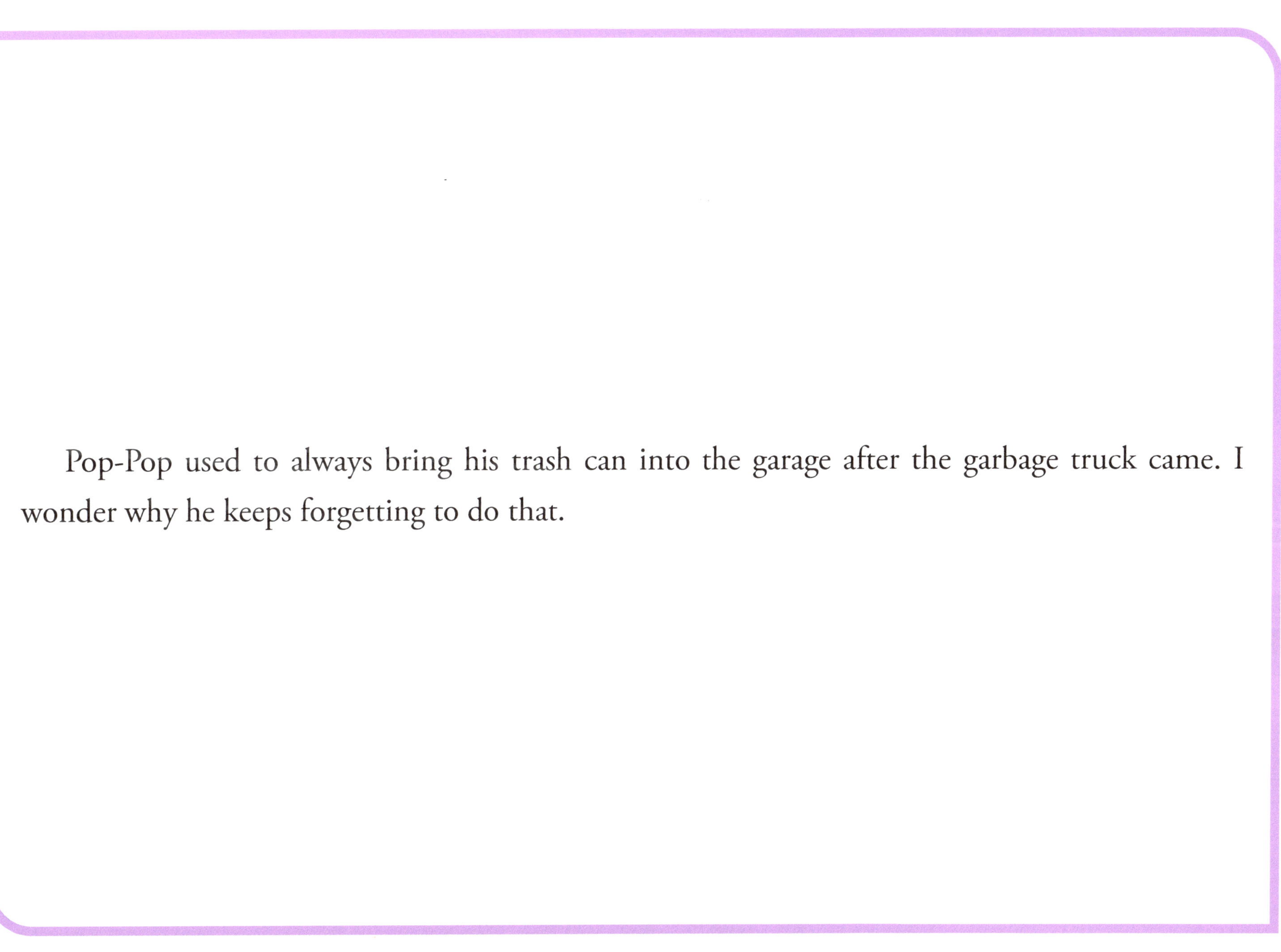

Pop-Pop used to always bring his trash can into the garage after the garbage truck came. I wonder why he keeps forgetting to do that.

I remember how Mom-Mom used to like to cook. I loved her meatballs! Did she forget how to make them? She does not make them anymore.

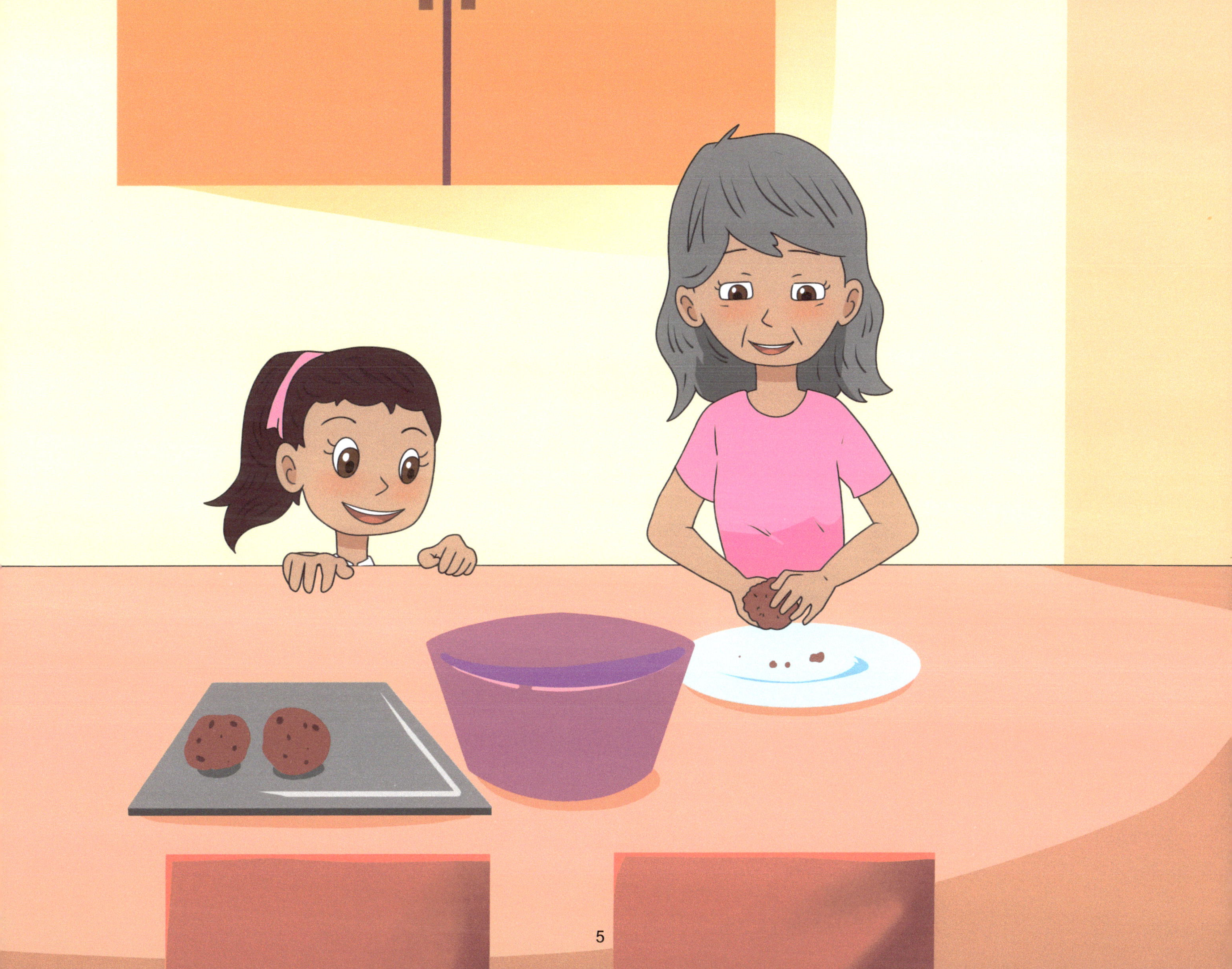

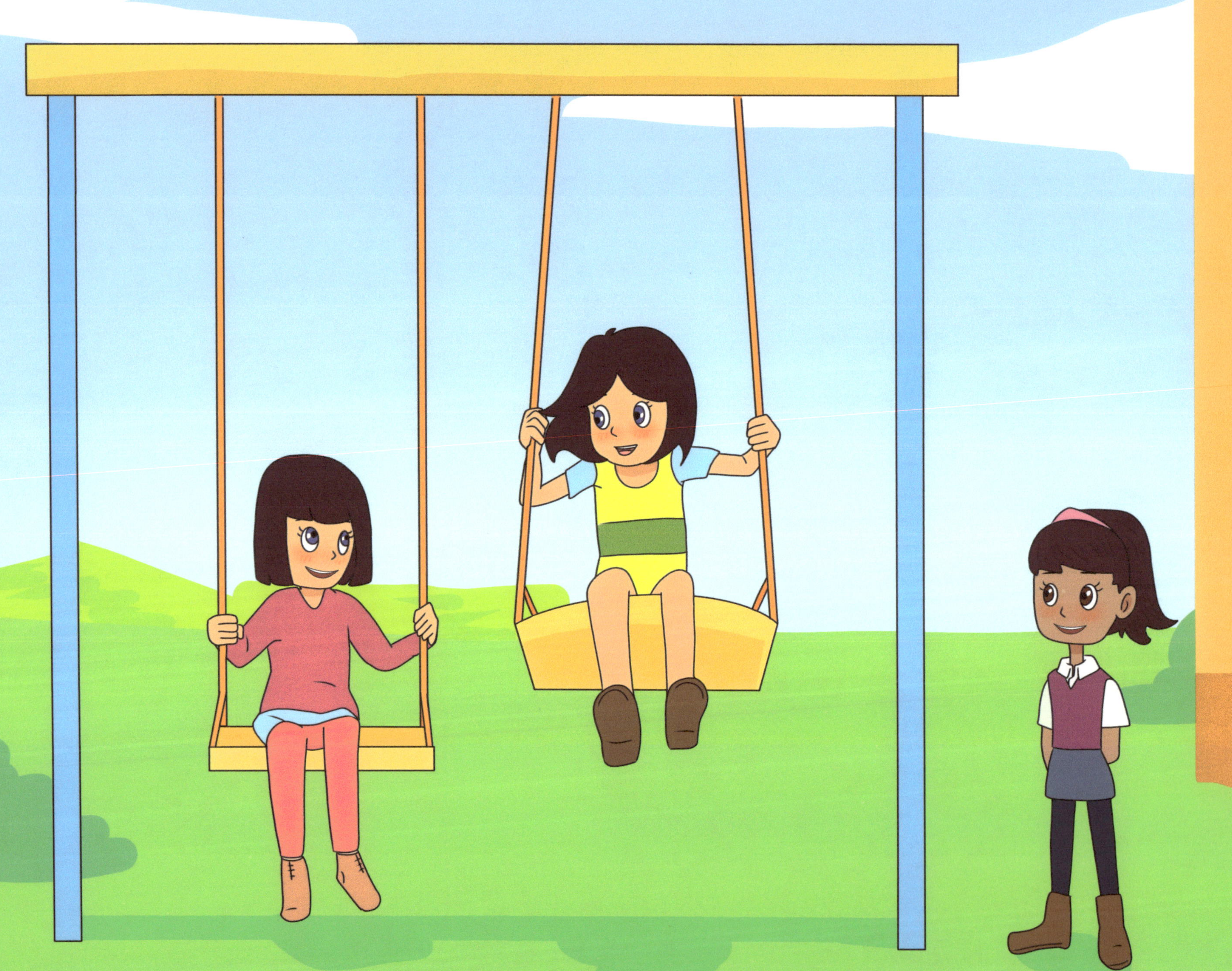

I want to know why when people get old, they forget stuff. I don't forget stuff. I forget to clean my room sometimes. Well, I don't really forget. I just don't feel like cleaning it, especially when my friends Lindsay and Jillian come over to play on the swings. They are my best friends. I wonder if I really did forget to clean my room. Would that mean I was getting old too?

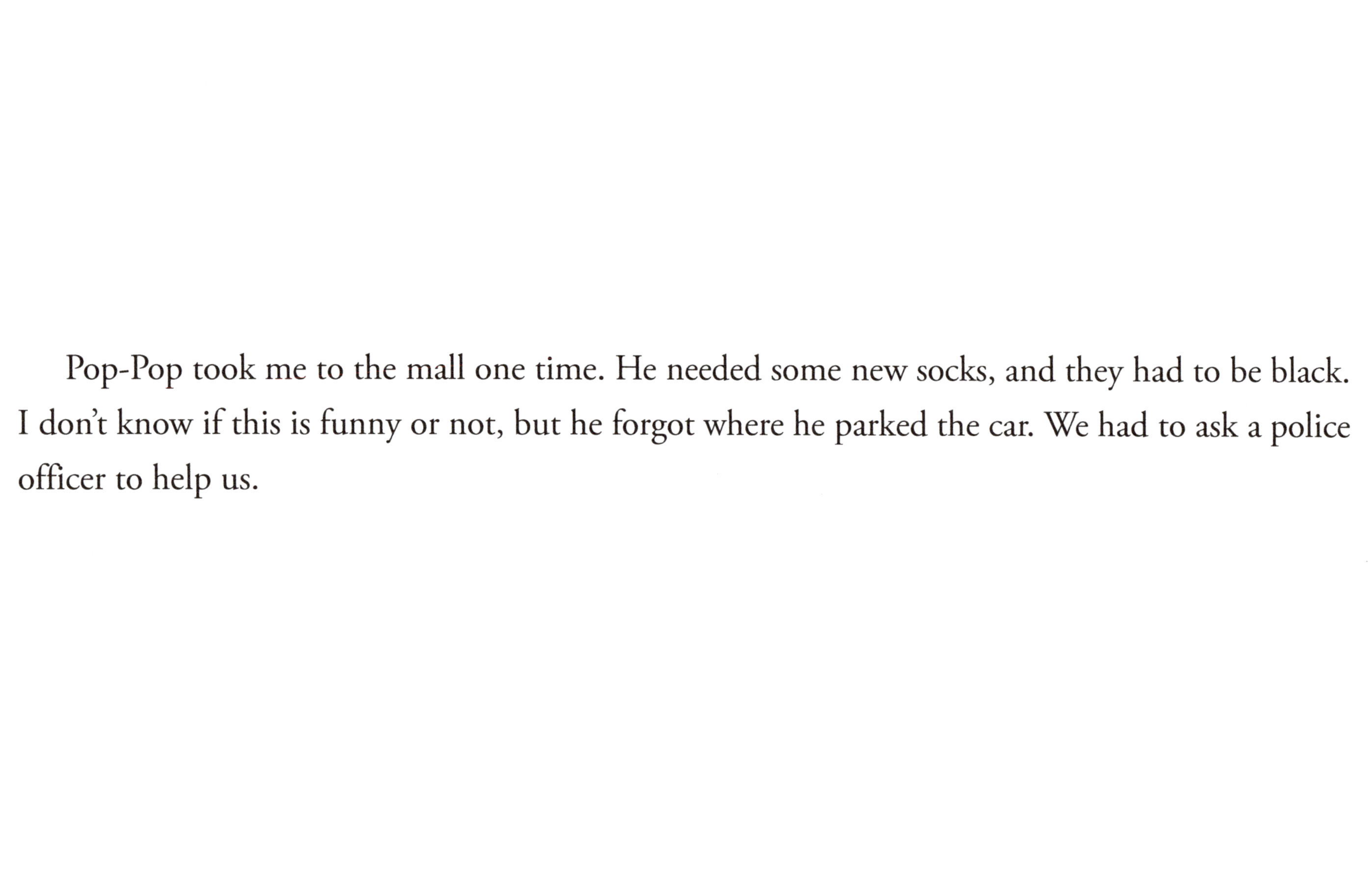

Pop-Pop took me to the mall one time. He needed some new socks, and they had to be black. I don't know if this is funny or not, but he forgot where he parked the car. We had to ask a police officer to help us.

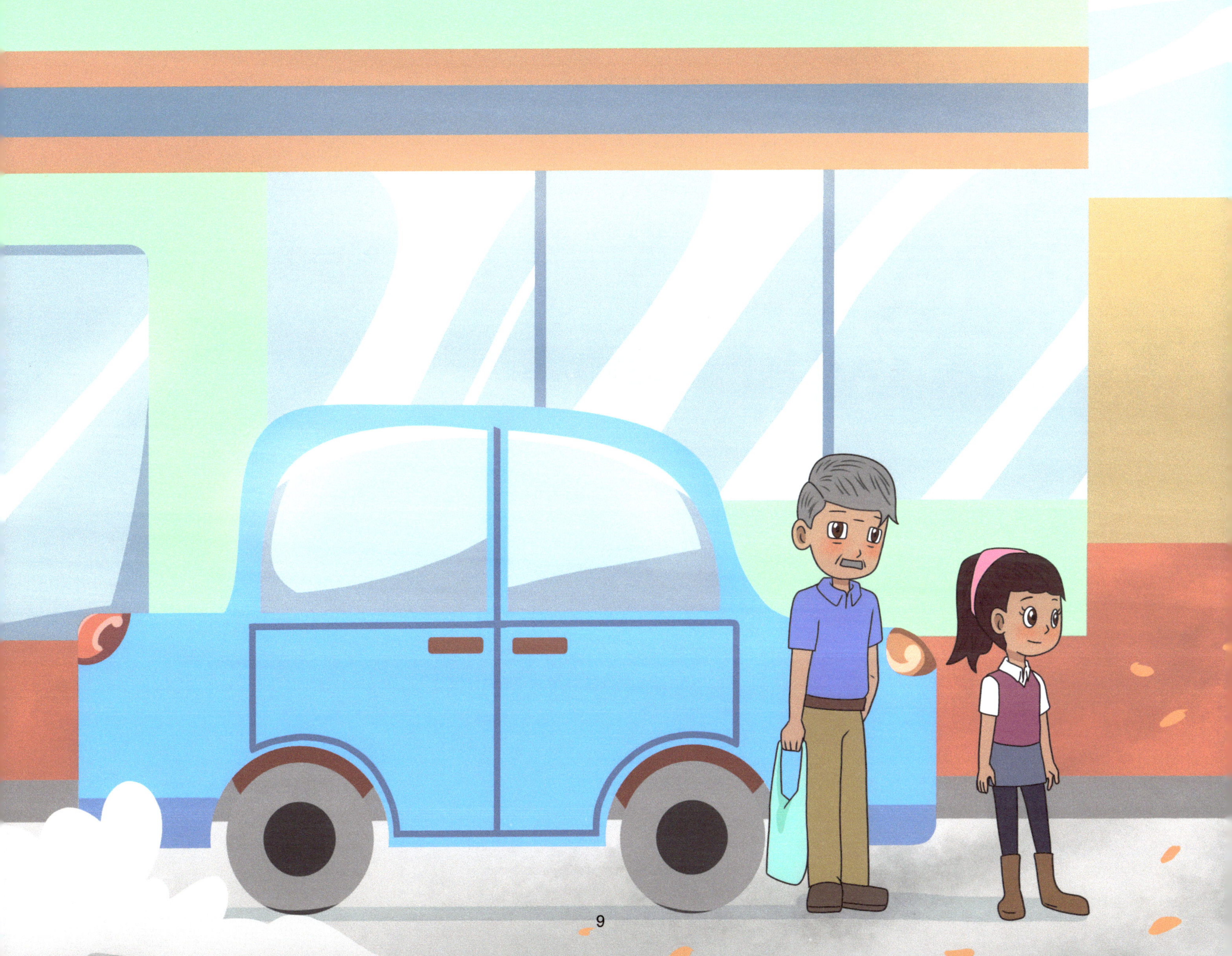

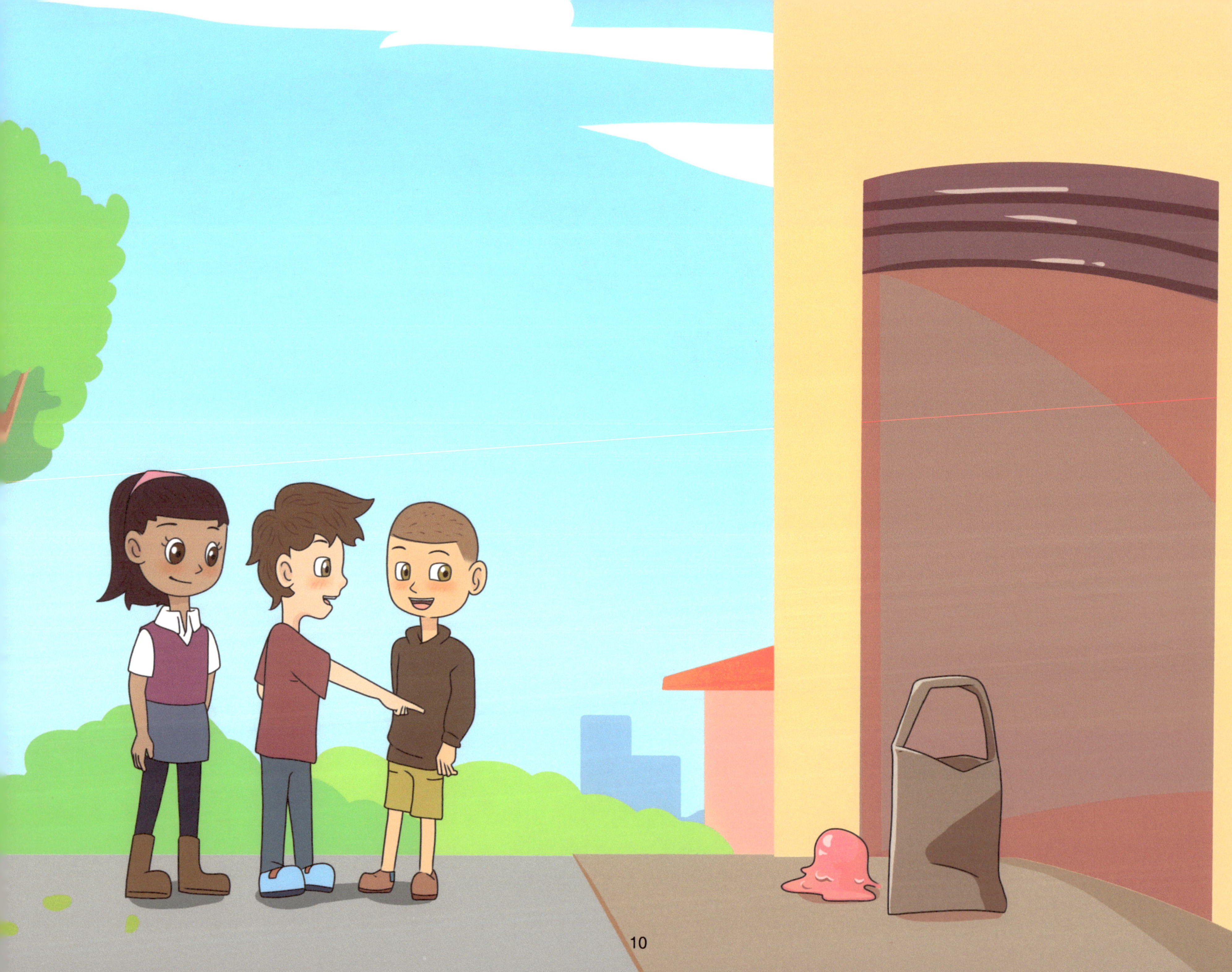

My friends Sean and James tell me their aunt Roseanna does funny forgetful stuff. She sometimes thinks that her house is not her house. Sometimes she tries to leave her house late at night by herself, but that's not funny. She once left her groceries in the garage, and the ice cream melted all over the floor. Now that's funny! Sean and James tell me she may have to go into some kind of home for assistance. I know they will miss her and visit her.

I wonder what I can do to help Mom-Mom and Pop-Pop. Maybe I can make them notes so they don't forget. My friend Gina's Mom-Mom and Pop-Pop don't forget like mine. Why is that?

My cousin Billy's Mom-Mom and Pop-Pop still go to work every day. They help out at the church, fixing and cleaning things to make the church look nice.

Sometimes people forget things because they are busy, right?

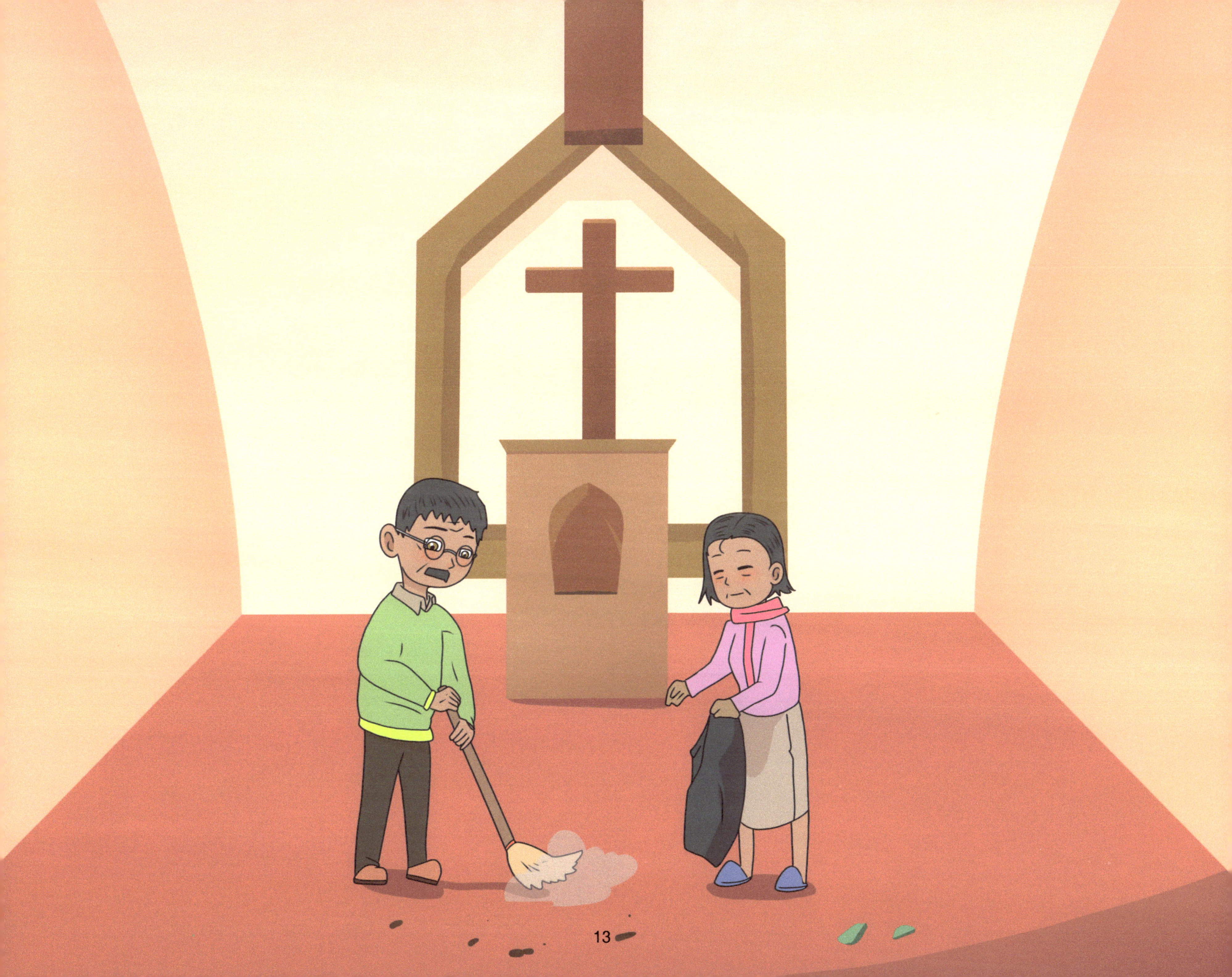

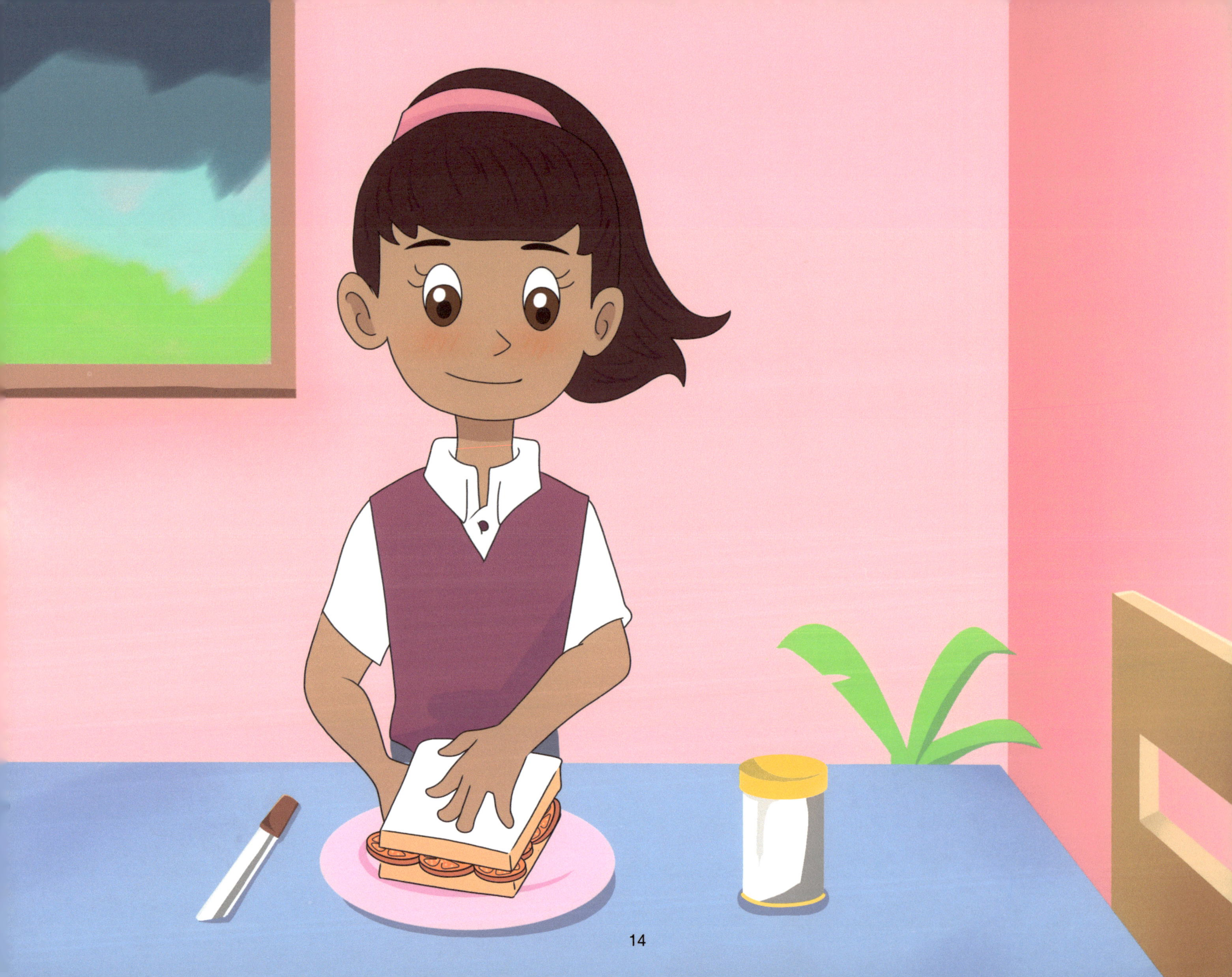

I can help Mom-Mom and Pop-Pop with things they need to do around the house. I can make them sandwiches for lunch. They sure do like cheese and tomato on white bread with a little bit of mayonnaise. Maybe Aunt Helen can help them with dinner. If our family helps and we do what we can, we can keep them from going into a home for assistance like Sean and James's aunt Roseanna, right?

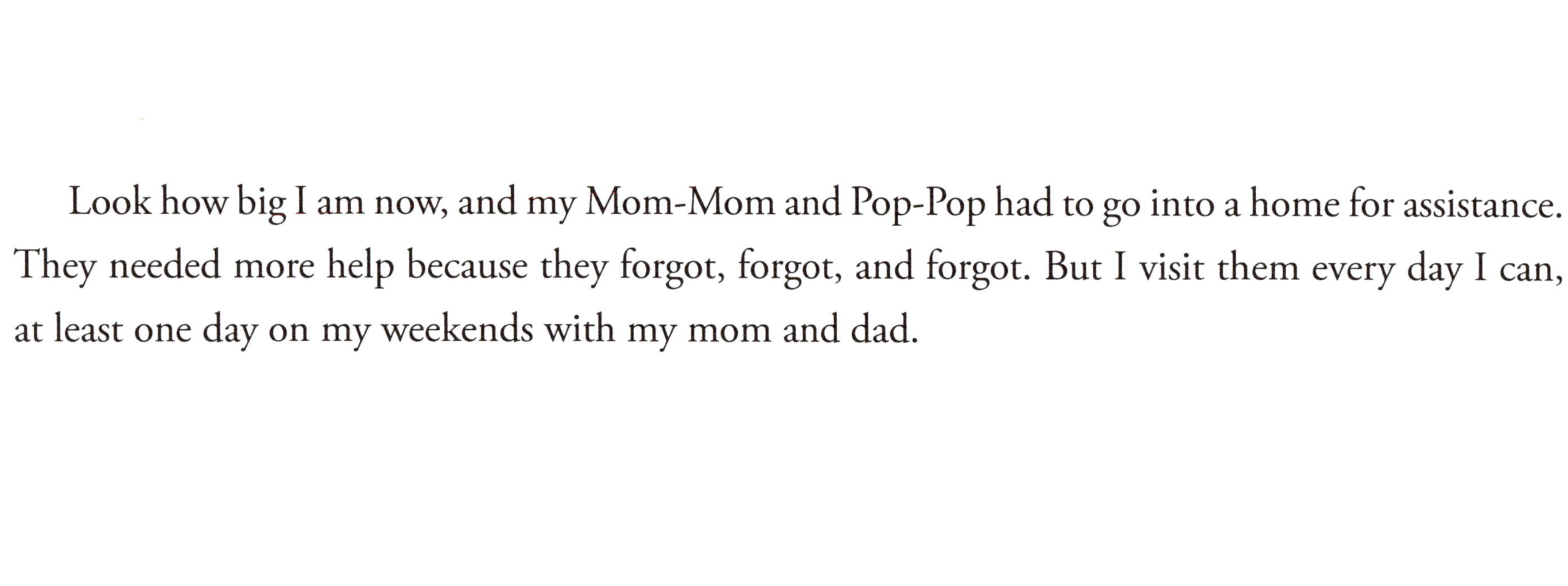

Look how big I am now, and my Mom-Mom and Pop-Pop had to go into a home for assistance. They needed more help because they forgot, forgot, and forgot. But I visit them every day I can, at least one day on my weekends with my mom and dad.

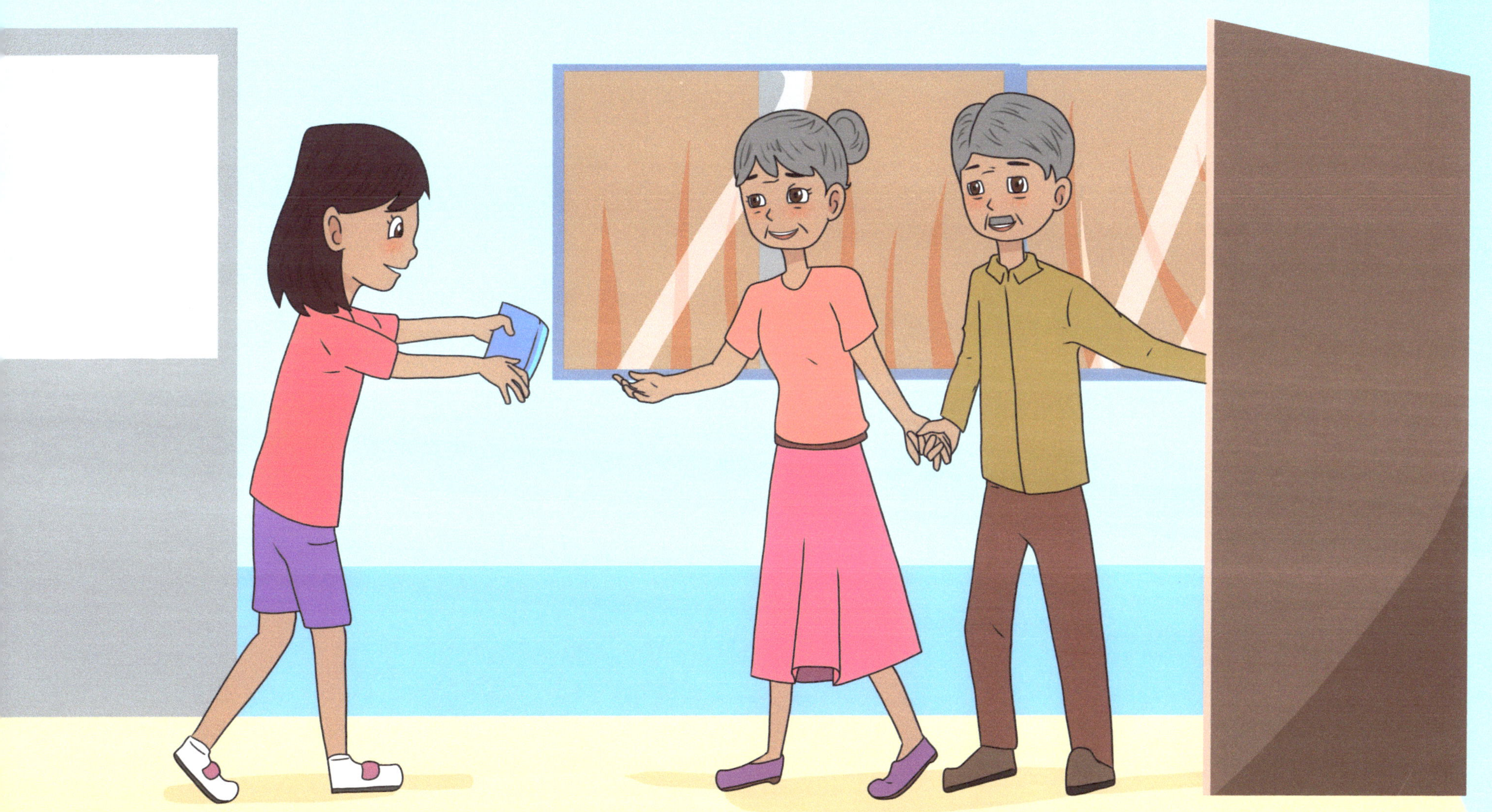

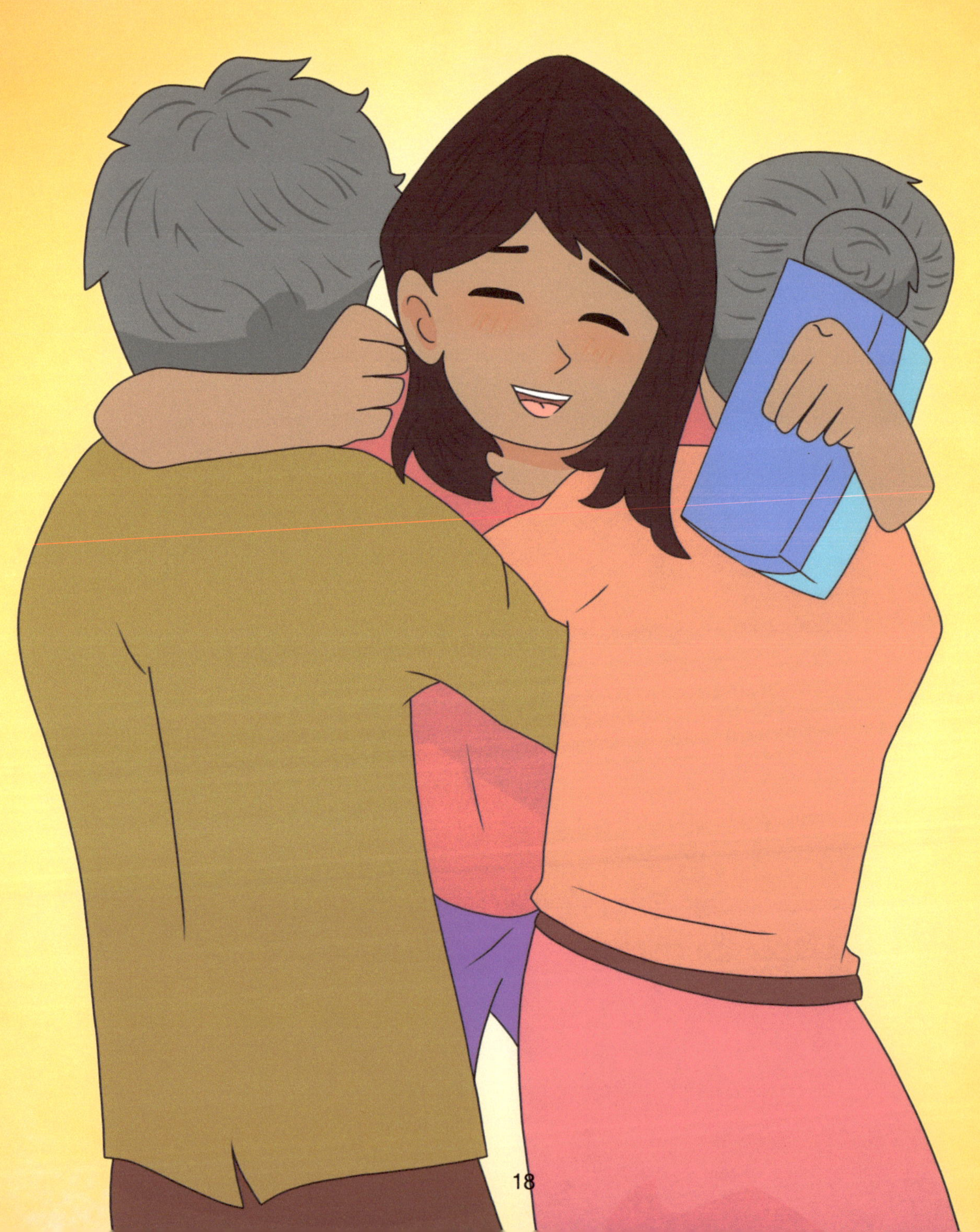

Mom-Mom and Pop-Pop give me hugs like they used to and tell me how much they love me. They like the new place where they live. I always bring them treats like they used to bring me when I was a smaller kid. I asked my Mom-Mom to give me her meatball recipe so I can make her meatballs like she use to make me. She giggles and smiles at me.

They decorate their new home for all the holidays, just like me. They play games, sing, and dance, just like me. I know they are getting older, and they are going to forget stuff. But they have made lots of friends and seem happy, but they're nowhere near as happy as when they see me.

When I go to visit my Mom-Mom and Pop-Pop, I start singing the same old song, and they join on in singing along…

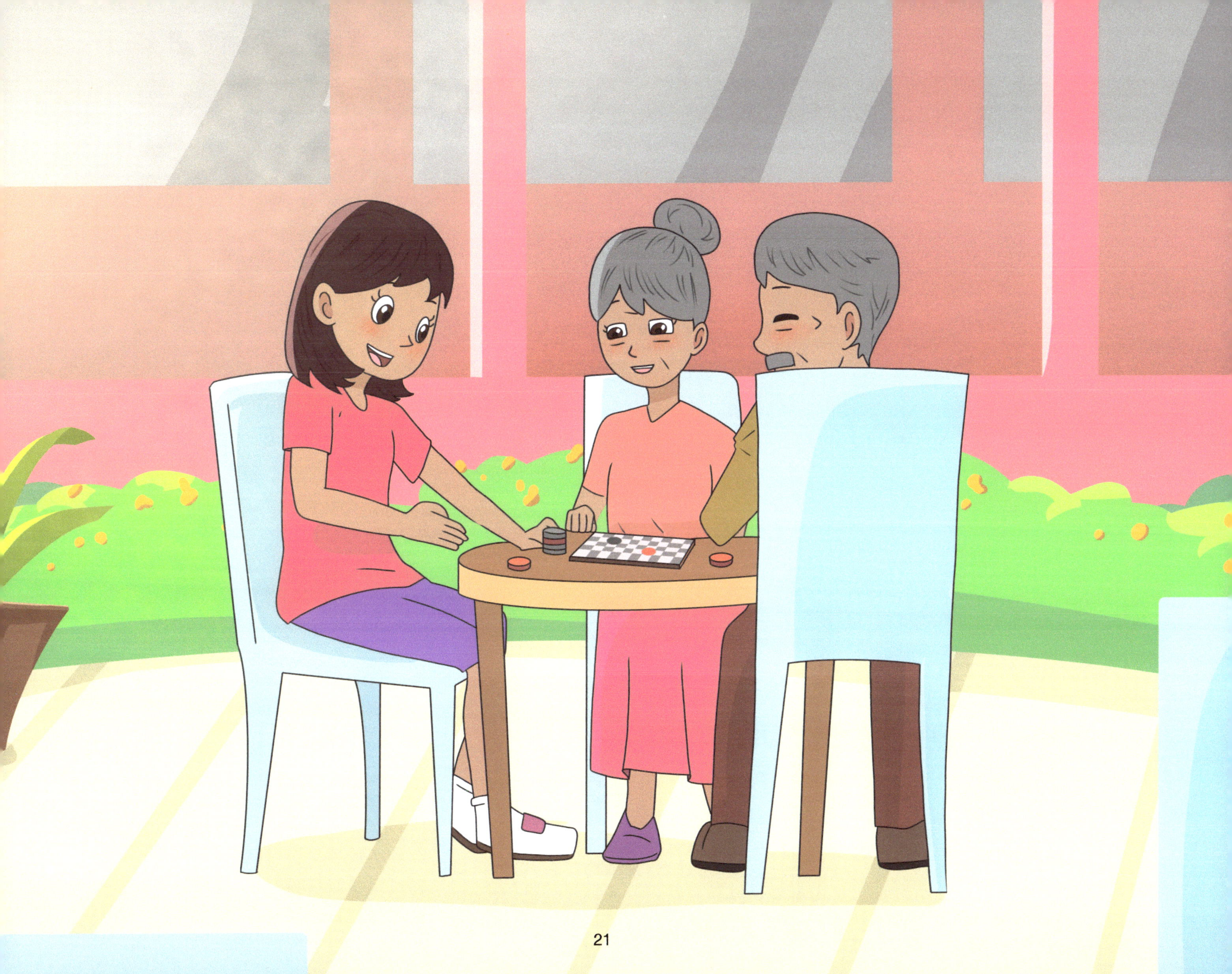

Each day I love to visit you

I sing to you,

"How do you do?"

Then you sing to me,

"I'm doing fine."

And you say to me,

"I have not seen you in some time,"

Even though I know

I was with you yesterday

I sing to you,

"How do you do?"

Then you sing to me,

"I'm doing fine."

About the Author

While concentrating most of her time on songwriting due to her love for country music since she was a young child, she found her way to creating stories about people in her life. She resides not too far from where she grew up in Bryn Mawr, Montgomery County. She now resides in Delaware County. She's a Delco girl, and some say she has the accent to prove it. She's very thankful for her two sons, her husband, and her entire family. She loves to laugh and loves to smile. Enjoy!